BREATHING BETTER

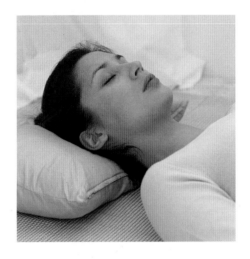

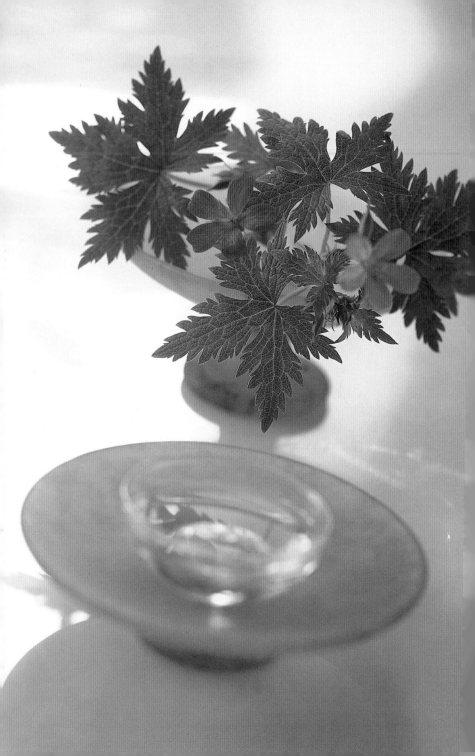

BREATHING
BETTER

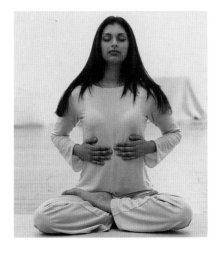

to beat ailments, combat allergies
and boost energy

RAJE AIREY

LORENZ BOOKS

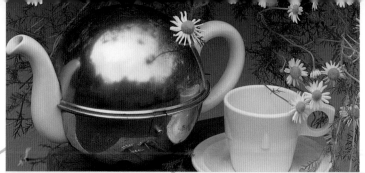

contents

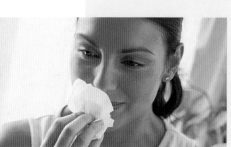

BREATHING BETTER

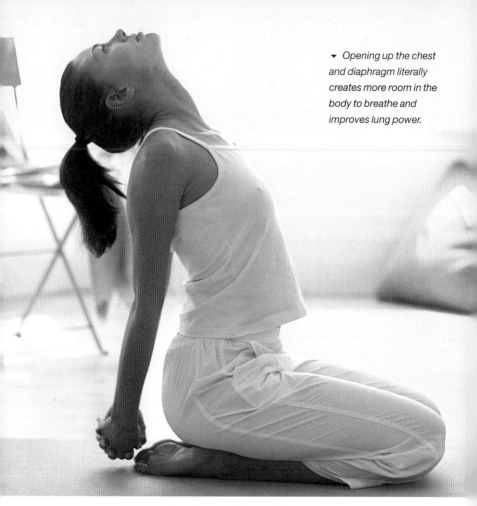

▼ Opening up the chest and diaphragm literally creates more room in the body to breathe and improves lung power.

introduction

To breathe is to be alive. From the moment we take our first breath until we finally expire, breathing is what connects each and every one of us to life. It is estimated that we breathe in and out nearly 25,000 times a day, yet research estimates that only one in ten of us breathes correctly, and that most of us use only a fraction of our lung capacity.

And that is before we take into account the worrying increase in the occurrence of respiratory diseases and disorders, particularly those that are allergy-related.

This book contains 50 natural, drug-free treatments designed to help you breathe better. Some of these are aimed at specific complaints while others are targeted towards increasing lung capacity, building immunity and improving resistance to allergies and infections. However, first it is useful to understand how breathing works and how it influences our health.

the respiratory system

The human body can go without food for weeks and without water for days, but without oxygen we cannot survive for more than a few minutes. The body's breathing apparatus is known as the respiratory system and is, together with the heart and blood supply, probably the most important system in the body. When working properly it extracts the oxygen from the air that we need to live and discharges carbon dioxide waste from the blood.

The respiratory system is made up of the ribcage, with its linking intercostal muscles, the diaphragm – a sheet of muscle between the chest and stomach – and the respiratory tract, which comprises the airways and lungs. When we breathe in the diaphragm contracts and moves down increasing the capacity of the chest cavity, and the muscles that link the ribs contract, pulling the ribs up and out. These two processes cause the lungs to expand. Air is drawn in through the nose where it is warmed and taken down into the lungs. When enough air has been inhaled (inspiration), the muscles and diaphragm relax, compressing the lungs, and the air is exhaled (expiration). Then the diaphragm contracts once more and the cycle

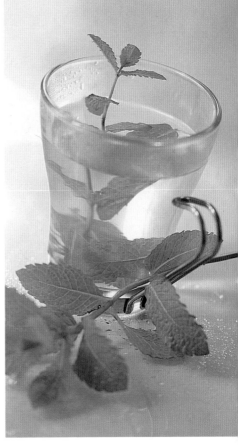

▲ Certain herbs, such as peppermint, can help to open up the airways.

begins again. After the air passes through the nose it enters the trachea (windpipe) and the bronchi, which are small airways that run through each lung. These bronchi become smaller and smaller, eventually taking the form of bronchioles, which end as tiny air sacs called alveoli. The alveoli are linked to blood capillaries that exchange oxygen and carbon dioxide at a very quick rate.

breathing rates

On average we take about 12 breaths per minute, according to the body's needs. If stressed, we tend to breathe at a faster rate, which can lead to muscle tension and eventually dizziness. Rapid breathing also occurs during strenuous exercise, an asthma attack or when frightened, because the body's need for oxygen increases. As the levels of oxygen and carbon dioxide return to normal, breathing resumes its usual slower rate. As we breathe normally and efficiently, the diaphragm contracts and becomes flat, increasing the space in the chest into which the lungs can expand. When the lungs are able to expand to their full capacity, all residual carbon dioxide is expelled and more oxygen can be inhaled.

breathing and health

The quality of our breathing affects our health in many different ways. Every cell in the body uses oxygen to extract the energy that's locked away in food, and our energy levels, mental powers, moods, creativity and emotional well-being all depend on the oxygen supply provided by our breathing. It is impossible to separate the health of our respiratory system from the rest of our lives, not only on a physical level, but also on mental and emotional levels.

Many ancient traditions have linked breathing with spiritual experience. The ancient Hebrews, for example, used the word "wind", the breath, in connection with the soul, and in India, "prana" or "spiritual breath" is seen as the life-force of the body's subtle energy system. So breathing affects our well-being at the level of mind, body and soul. It is our connection with the universe: trees and plants take in the carbon dioxide we exhale and replace it with life-giving oxygen in a cycle of integration and wholeness.

COMMON BREATHING PROBLEMS

The pressures of modern living have created an almost breathless culture. As we struggle to keep up with the fast pace of life, we become tense and anxious. This creates shallow and restricted breathing patterns, which lead to a tendency to over-breathe as we gulp in mouthfuls of air to compensate.

Furthermore, a variety of disorders – including physical injury, poor posture, infections, viruses, allergies and chronic disease – can disrupt and endanger the normal breathing process. Most breathing disorders are made worse by environmental pollution, or even by what we eat and drink, and in the case of allergies these can be the sole cause. Cigarette smoke also causes breathing problems, increasing the incidence of serious diseases such as lung cancer and emphysema.

Other disorders, ranging from the common cold, bronchitis and pleurisy to life-threatening conditions such as pneumonia and TB, are the result of bacterial or viral infections, which are made more likely by a weak immune system.

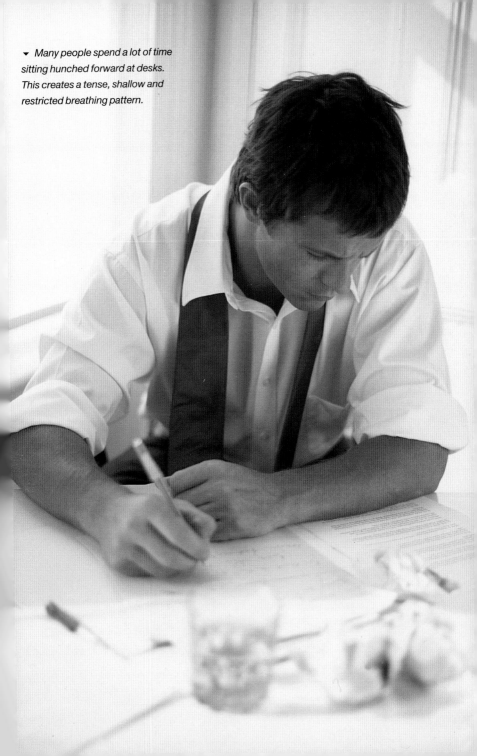

▼ Many people spend a lot of time sitting hunched forward at desks. This creates a tense, shallow and restricted breathing pattern.

breathing therapies

Whether our breathing problems are related to chronic asthma or bronchitis, or to allergies such as hay fever and rhinitis, or even the common cold, there are countless ways that we can improve our breathing. The following pages present 50 natural, drug-free methods, some of which offer short-term quick-fix solutions, while others take a longer-term view. All, however, are based on holistic principles, recognizing that good health is achieved when mind, body and soul are balanced and in harmony.

The treatments are drawn from a variety of natural healing traditions, and include methods to re-educate our breathing as well as remedies and exercises that will rebalance, calm and strengthen it. Complementary therapies such as aromatherapy, shiatsu, homeopathy and reiki healing are included, as well as yoga, herbal remedies, dietary advice, and lifestyle recommendations. We hope that you will find something here that works for you.

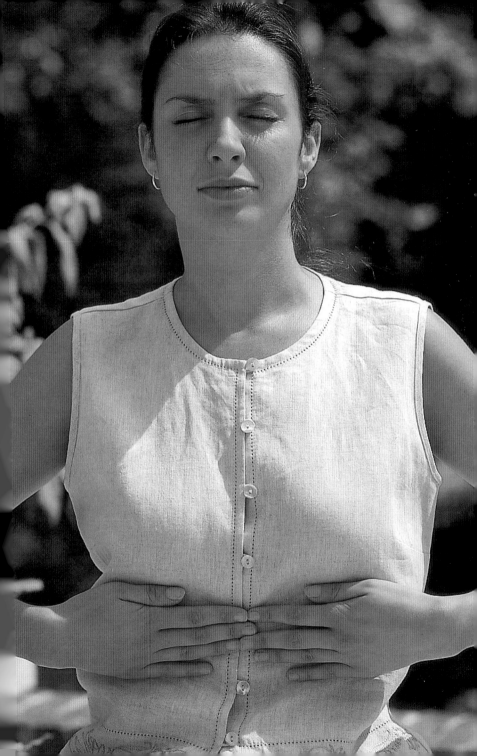

1

Buteyko method

Konstantin Buteyko (1923–2003), a Russian doctor, pioneered a theory and method of breathing that claims to be one of the most effective natural treatments for asthma and breathing disorders.

According to Buteyko, many breathing problems and disorders are linked to over-breathing, or hyperventilation, which causes an excessive reduction in the body's levels of carbon dioxide (CO_2).

health and carbon dioxide
Carbon dioxide is not only found in the atmosphere, but also in the alveoli (air sacs) in our lungs. Low levels of CO_2 in the body cause blood vessels to spasm (as happens in an asthma attack) so that oxygen is not properly absorbed by the body's tissues and vital organs. CO_2 is also involved in

regulating the body's pH balance; insufficient CO_2 shifts the body towards alkalinity, which in turn has a weakening effect on the immune system, making it much more susceptible to viruses and allergies.

the Buteyko test
It is possible to measure your CO_2 level: breathe out, hold your nose and then count in seconds until you need to breathe in. A count of 60 corresponds to a level of 6.5 per cent CO_2 in the lungs and perfect health; between 40–50 is good, less than 30 indicates health problems, and if you have severe to moderate asthma, you may not be able to hold for more than 5–10 seconds.

self-help measure
Try to make an effort to breathe only through your nose, if possible. Buteyko practitioners claim that this practice alone can reduce asthma symptoms by up to 50 per cent.

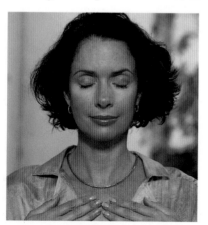

◄ *The Buteyko method is based on retraining our breathing so that we take a longer pause at the end of the out-breath.*

2

alternate nostril breathing

When our breathing is calm and steady we are more able to think clearly. Calming and regulating the breathing is one of the best methods for stress reduction and improving concentration.

Our emotional state is reflected by our breathing patterns. So, if we are feeling nervous or under strain, we may tend to hyperventilate (over-breathe) or to inhale very short and shallow breaths.

The yoga technique that is known as alternate nostril breathing is designed to calm the nervous system, as well as harmonize the left and right sides of the brain. This also helps to redress any imbalance between introvert and extrovert tendencies – between an overactive mind that is draining our physical energies and an overexcited nervous system that is making us confused and mentally exhausted. It will also help clear blocked sinuses, so have some tissues handy.

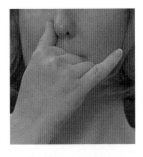

1 Two breaths form one round: do several rounds while sitting in an upright, comfortable position. Place your thumb at the base of your right nostril and pinch it closed. Breathe in through the left nostril.

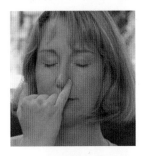

2 Relax your thumb and position your little finger at the base of the left nostril and pinch it closed. Breathe out through your right nostril. Your breathing will deepen slowly and naturally so don't force it.

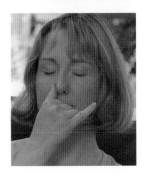

3 Now breathe in on the right, then close that nostril again and breathe out on the left. Continue to breathe slowly and steadily through alternate nostrils, using your thumb and finger to close the nostrils.

3

stretching and expanding

Expanding the chest enables the lungs to fill more efficiently with air, which will in turn bring more oxygen to all the cells in the body, including the respiratory organs.

Chronic tension and anxiety can lead to restricted muscles, so that it becomes difficult to relax the diaphragm and breathe properly. Many asthmatics are tight around the diaphragm area, which exacerbates breathing difficulties. The following exercise is particularly good for asthma and other chest problems. When done on a regular basis, they will help improve breathing and

blood flow to the chest muscles and lungs and help to open up the chest. First of all, stand with your feet hip-width apart, arms by your sides. Slowly taking a deep breath in, raise your arms out to the sides. Still breathing in, raise your arms up over your head, rising up on to your toes. Breathing out, drop your arms and return to standing. Then repeat this sequence twice more.

chest expansion

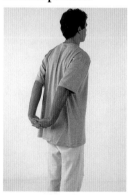

1 Stand with your feet hip-width apart and your knees slightly bent. Clasp your hands behind your back.

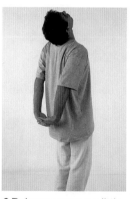

2 Raise your arms a little, leaning back slightly. Then lean forwards as far as possible, bending from the hips.

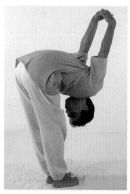

3 Raise your arms and keep them as high as is comfortable. Slowly straighten up, relax and repeat twice more.

4 making sounds

Singing, humming and playing a wind instrument
are all excellent examples of how making sounds
can help to strengthen our lungs and improve
our breathing.

Playing a wind instrument (such as a flute or recorder) or singing is an effective way of improving your lung function and can really help counter hyperventilation. When you play a wind instrument, you are training yourself to control your breathing to produce the longest phrases. Singers also have to learn to control their breathing, so that they breathe in at an appropriate point in the song. If you feel too shy to sing in front of others, then practise when you are alone – in the shower or in the car, for example.

sound meditations

Combining sound with meditation is another way of improving lung capacity; it also has the advantage of quietening the mind and emotions. Try the following methods.

bee-breath meditation

This is a relaxing technique that is best done last thing at night to aid a good night's sleep.

Sit in an upright but relaxed position and close your eyes. Keeping your mouth closed, take a breath in. On the out-breath, start to make a humming sound, repeating the sound each time you breathe out. Keep your mind focused on the sound and let it become louder each time, so that you sound like a humming bee.

om-sound breathing

Sitting comfortably, inhale deeply and vocalize the sounds "ah", "oo" and "mm" as you exhale, joining them together to make the sound of "om". In the East, this is a sacred sound, the vibrations of which are said to heal and balance body, mind and spirit.

▾ Combining sound with meditation is a useful technique for calming our breathing.

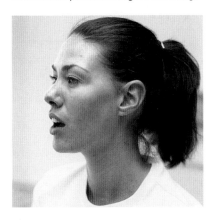

5 breathing exercises

To breathe is to be inspired. Breathing brings life-giving oxygen to the body and cleanses our system of impurities. Breathing exercises help to rebalance our breathing patterns.

Regulating your breathing helps you to feel calm and centred in body and mind. Try the simple control exercise seen here. There are also many yoga exercises, known as "pranayama", that are based on working with the breath. The cleansing exercise shown below has a powerful mucus-clearing action and so is ideal for those who suffer from allergies, a blocked nose or sinus trouble. The exercise also strengthens the muscles of the abdomen, is good for a sluggish digestive system, and may even give your skin a healthy glow.

easy breath control exercise

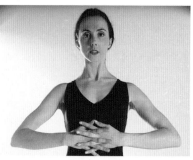

1 Place your hands with your palms under your chest, on your ribs, and your fingers loosely interlocked. Inhale slowly and continuously through your nose to a count of four. Stay relaxed.

2 As you inhale, concentrate on letting your ribs expand laterally; your fingers should gently part. Don't let your ribs jut forward. Exhale slowly, expelling all the breath from your lungs. Repeat.

cleansing breath routine

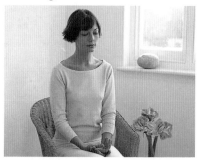

1 Sitting with your head up and your back straight, breathe out in a series of short, sharp exhalations through the nose. Tighten your stomach muscles and squeeze the air out of your lungs.

2 Relax your stomach muscles – you will automatically inhale. After the tenth in-breath, breathe out for as long as you can and try to empty the lungs. Take a few resting breaths and do another set.

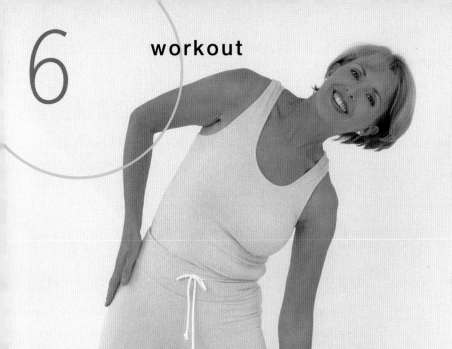

Prevention is better than cure. Aerobic exercise builds stamina, strengthens the immune system, and opens up the breathing. Try it and feel your body pulsate with life.

7 swimming

A session at your local pool provides one of the best types of exercise for strengthening the lungs, opening the chest and coordinating the breathing. It can help a wide range of breathing problems.

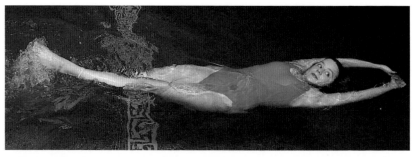

▲ The benefits of swimming are well known. As well as being a good all-round form of exercise, it is especially helpful for regulating breathing disorders by reducing stress and tension and opening up the chest and diaphragm. Backstroke is particularly beneficial.

Swimming is widely accepted as being a highly effective all-round form of exercise for the whole body. Its rhythmical actions encourage deeper breathing, increase lung capacity and improve the body's blood supply.

Regular sessions at the pool benefit the circulatory and respiratory systems and help to improve mobility in the joints and muscles, thus increasing muscular strength and tone. The immune system also gets a boost, making this form of exercise helpful for easing all kinds of conditions, including chronic breathing problems such as asthma.

Swimming can lessen the effects of stress and tension, which can produce tight or "held" patterns of breathing. If you have bronchitis or severe asthma, you may not be able to swim for long, but take it gently and you will gradually improve.

AQUA YOGA
Neatly uniting the benefits of yoga and swimming, aqua yoga combines slow stretching with breathing and relaxation techniques. Bodies feel virtually weightless in water, so more effective stretches can be achieved without the risk of strain.

T'ai chi

In China, the non-combative martial arts system called T'ai chi is very much a part of daily life. Its gentle, meditative movements ease stress and help to deepen and regulate breathing.

Breathing techniques dominate the routine shown here, but any T'ai chi routine can improve breathing, by virtue of its ability to ease stress. Keep the moves flowing and slow, and co-ordinated with your breath.

four-directional breathing

1 Stand with your feet apart and knees slightly bent. As you inhale, bring your hands, palms face-up, to chest height.

2 As you exhale, turn the palms to face away from you and extend your arms as if pushing something away.

3 On the next inhalation, turn your palms back to face your body. Soften and relax your arms and draw them back in towards your chest.

4 Exhale, turning the palms out and extending your arms to your sides.

5 Inhale and bring your arms in towards your chest again.

6 On the next out-breath, turn your palms face-up and reach up towards the sky.

7 Inhale and let your arms descend, palms face-down.

8 As your hands and arms pass below your navel, begin breathing out and push downwards with your hands, sending the energy towards the earth.

On the next inhalation, bring your hands up to begin a new cycle of four breaths. Repeat the sequence several times.

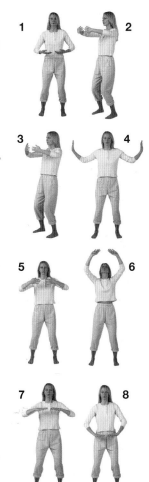

9 Alexander technique

Better breathing is made easier by the Alexander technique, a system of body awareness that works to correct "patterns of misuse" in the body's balance and structure.

Poor posture is linked to many breathing disorders. For instance, asthmatics often round their back and shoulders and thrust their neck forwards. Over time, this builds up into a pattern of muscular tension which is difficult to correct.

Developed by F M Alexander in the early 20th century, the Alexander technique is a system of re-educating the body to bring it back into alignment. It focuses in particular on the dynamic relationship between the head, neck and back which are usually out of alignment.

The Alexander technique focuses on teaching how to perform simple movements – such as sitting and walking – correctly. It can be especially helpful for breathing disorders caused or exacerbated by poor posture and stress.

walking with awareness

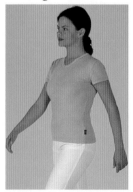

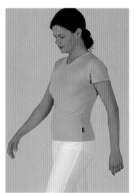

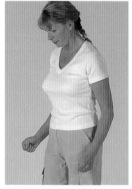

To walk correctly, the head should lead the movement. The spine is straight, and the arms hang loosely at the sides.

Here the the alignment between head, neck and back has been lost and the head has dropped at the neckline.

In this example, the shoulders are hunched and the arms are tense. The head is down when it should be held high.

10 yoga postures

Based on postures and breathwork, yoga can help with many breathing problems, as well as strengthening the immune system and building resistance to allergy and infection. ✦

Yoga is both calming and energizing. Practised regularly it helps to increase stamina and flexibility, and also encourages the body to release patterns of tension and tightness. It does not matter how fit or flexible you are; the important thing while practising yoga (as with any form of exercise) is to work within your capabilities and not to strain or over-exert yourself in an attempt to achieve the "perfect" posture.

bridge pose

Lie flat on your back, arms by your sides. Bend your knees, feet hip-width apart, just in front of the buttocks. On an in-breath, lift your pelvis and raise your back so that you "stand" on your feet and shoulders. Breathe normally. On an out-breath, slowly lower yourself to the floor so that your buttocks reach the floor last.

simplified camel pose

Sit on your heels with your hands clasped behind you and breathe in. On the out-breath, drop your head back and raise your arms a little. Breathe for a few seconds, then return to an upright position on an out-breath. Repeat three or four times.

▾ *The "bridge pose" expands the ribcage and can be helpful in encouraging the expulsion of mucus.*

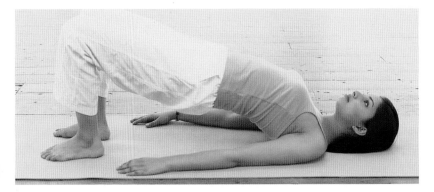

11

stretching with a partner

Gentle stretching exercises are a good way of opening the chest. Having a partner to help you stretch can be effective when you are suffering from mild breathing difficulties.

During episodes of mild asthma or bronchitis, working with a partner can feel very supportive. The following stretching exercises will ease muscular tension in the ribcage and encourage the chest to open.

stretching the lungs
This sequence of three stretches can help to counter the forward-bending hunched posture typical of someone with a shallow, rapid breathing pattern or congestive problems.

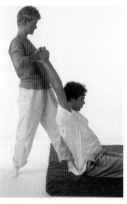

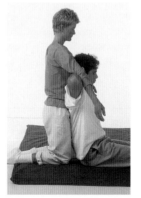

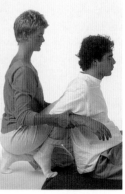

1 Sit your partner on the floor with legs straight. Stand behind, one foot in front of the other, and put the side of your leg against the spine. Take their hands, gripping the thumbs, and as you both exhale, lift up and lean back until your partner feels the stretch.

2 Kneel down behind your partner and ask them to clasp their hands behind their neck. Bring your arms in front of your partner's arms, and on the out-breath gently open up their elbows to the sides. Your partner should feel their chest opening.

3 Bring one knee up to support your partner's lower back and take hold of their lower arms. On the out-breath, bring their elbows towards each other, stretching to the middle of their back.

12 back massage

The soothing pressure of a back massage is an effective treatment for relaxing the diaphragm, easing congestion in the airways and encouraging the expulsion of excess mucus.

Excess mucus production is associated with many breathing disorders, from a viral infection such as a cold, to allergic symptoms associated with hay fever or the persistent "plugs" of mucus that block the airways in asthma and bronchitis.

simple three-step back massage

Make sure your partner is lying on a firm, but comfortable, surface and that the room is warm and draught-free. Keep their lower body covered with a towel or blanket as you work. You may like to use a little massage oil, such as sweet almond.

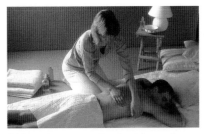

2 Move to your partner's side, and using the whole of your hand, pull up steadily, one hand after the other, working all the way up and down one side of your partner's back a few times. Repeat on the other side.

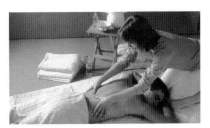

1 Position yourself at your partner's head and use a smooth stroking movement, down either side of the spine, with your thumbs. Take your hands to the side and glide back up to the shoulders.

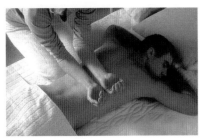

3 Stretch the back, by pressing your forearms and gliding them in opposite directions. As you work try to keep a steady pressure, lifting your arms when they reach the neck and buttocks. Return to the centre of the back and repeat twice more.

13

shiatsu massage

Stress and tension are associated with a shallow, rapid breathing pattern. A shiatsu massage can help to promote deeper, calmer breathing and so aid relaxation.

Shiatsu, like acupressure, works on the body's subtle energy system, which runs through the body along energy pathways, known as "meridians". By applying a firm pressure on meridian points, the flow of "chi" – the body's vital force – is stimulated. It also uses passive stretching movements to open up the body and ease tension.

Try the following as a good general technique. Put one hand just below your partner's sternum (breastbone) and slide the other hand, at the same level, under their back. Focus on this area and ask your partner to breathe into it. Slowly feel tension go and the muscles relax as the breath's healing energy reaches this area. Your partner's breathing should deepen and soften.

opening up the chest

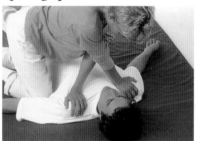

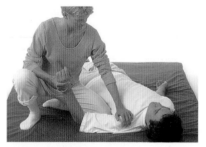

1 Have your partner lie flat on their back on a firm, but comfortable, surface. Kneeling at their side, cross your arms over and place your palms on your partner's shoulders. Ask your partner to breathe in, and on the out-breath bring your body weight over your hands, stimulating the first point of the lung meridian and gently opening the chest. Repeat three times.

2 Keep your left hand on your partner's shoulder and take a firm hold of their hand with your right hand. Lift the arm from the floor, shake it out and allow it to relax. Finally, hold on to your partner's thumb, and still holding the shoulder, give the arm and the lung meridian a good stretch.

14 rolfing

Breathing disorders are often associated with poor posture. Rolfing is a type of massage that aims to realign the body by working with its connective tissue.

Rolfing was developed by Dr Ida Rolf (1896–1979), an American biochemist. It aims to realign the body so that it can move in harmony with the forces of gravity. When the body structure is correctly balanced, we experience improved health and well-being.

Rolfing uses deep tissue massage to remould the body's connective tissue. While the technique can be rather painful at times, this is usually temporary and can be completely outweighed by the relief from chronic pain and discomfort caused by poor postural alignment. Although rolfing is not aimed at specific conditions, it has helped many asthma sufferers, as well as those suffering painful muscular conditions.

Rolfing often does more than simply remedy the body's structural problems, however. It is an holistic form of treatment that works on the whole person: body, mind and emotions. It recognizes that most physical problems also have a mental and emotional component. Problems with the lungs and respiration are often seen in people who have difficulties with letting go of painful experiences, especially those that happened a long time ago. When we are unable to process these experiences properly, it is as though they become "trapped" or stored in the body tissue and our system becomes clogged with "emotional junk". Consequently, during a rolfing treatment, manipulating deep-seated muscular tension can very often provoke an emotional release, such as crying or shouting.

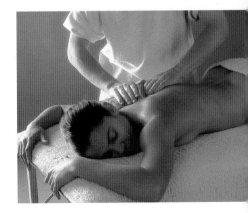

▸ Rolfing is a form of deep tissue massage that helps to release tension and improve breathing patterns.

15 osteopathy

Based on a series of manipulative techniques, osteopathy aims to realign the body's structure. It has been used to remedy many chronic respiratory conditions.

Osteopathy was founded by American doctor Andrew Still (1828-1917). It looks back to the fourth-century BC Hippocratic school of medical thought, in that it stresses the essential unity of all body parts and the body's innate self-healing mechanism.

Still identified the musculoskeletal system as a key element of health. Although we stand upright, our anatomy is still basically that of a creature which moves on all fours, and there is a constant strain on the whole framework. He recognized that the effect of gravity is particularly severe on the spine and that misalignment of the body's structure compromises health.

Osteopathy uses manipulative techniques that treat the whole body. These range from gentle, repeated movements of the joints to increase their mobility, to quick thrusting movements that rapidly guide the joint through its normal range. These latter manipulations often cause the clicking noise that many people experience during a session. An osteopathic treatment may also be accompanied by deep tissue massage.

Osteopathy works on the body's structure, so it can help redress postural problems linked to chronic breathing problems. These include a rounded back and shoulders and "collapsed" chest, as well as tightness around the intercostal muscles. It can also help with the back pain that many chronic asthma and bronchitis sufferers experience as a secondary symptom of their condition.

▲ During a treatment, the osteopath uses a series of manipulations to realign the body. This can help ease breathing problems.

16 reflexology

Also known as "zone therapy", reflexology can be helpful for a range of respiratory conditions. It works by stimulating specific pressure points on the feet or hands.

Reflexology is based on the idea that areas on the feet are linked along invisible nerve channels or energy pathways to different organs and systems of the rest of the body. By working on the appropriate area of the feet, it is possible to affect the respiratory system.

the chest reflex points

The ball of each foot represents either side of the chest and is where the reflex points to the respiratory system are found. The whole area is bounded by the diaphragm, the reflex that lies across the base of the ball of each foot.

breathing relief

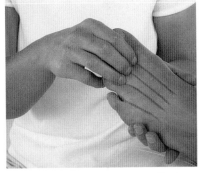

2 Fingerwalk the same area on the top of the feet to stimulate the chest lymph; this should encourage the removal of toxins.

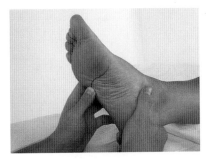

3 To relax the diaphragm, use a pressing movement with your thumb along the diaphragm line (the boundary where the ball of the foot meets the instep).

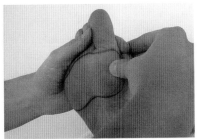

1 Using a firm thumb pressure, work the whole chest area to relieve congestion in the chest and lungs.

17

acupressure

By applying pressure to certain points on the body, it is possible to ease congestion in the lungs and sinuses, open up the airways and reduce symptoms of stress and tension.

Acupressure, which is based on very similar principles to shiatsu, uses finger pressure to stimulate and rebalance the energy flow along these meridians. It can be a useful quick-fix treatment that you can do on yourself (or with a partner) whenever you have a spare moment.

anxiety calmer

Rapid, shallow breathing or a tense "held-in" breath are often connected with anxiety and panic. In acupressure, there is a point known as the "Palace of Anxiety" that is located near the base of the thumb. Pressing into this point will have a calming and relaxing effect and should help your breathing to slow down and deepen.

self-treatment for sinus relief

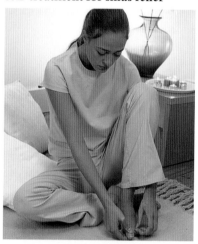

To relieve sinus congestion it can be helpful to work on foot acupressure points. Squeeze and press the tips of your toes and press and slide down their sides to the pads beneath. Continue this pressure, particularly on the big toes. To relieve a frontal sinus headache, apply pressure to just below the nail of the big toe.

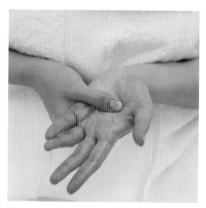

▲ *Pressing into the pressure point near the base of the thumb can release tension.*

Bring the scent of forest pine
into your home – add a
few drops of the essential oil
to a vaporizer and
enjoy a quick-fix treatment
to unblock a stuffy nose.

aromatic compress

Essential oils can have a dramatic influence on the respiratory system. A compress is a good way to use them without the risk of irritating the delicate mucous membranes.

Inhalation is one of the fastest ways of using essential oils, but it is not always well tolerated, especially when the nasal passages and bronchi are inflamed and irritated. There are many essential oils that can help with hay fever, rhinitis and allergic asthma. Some of the most gentle, but still effective, include camomile and lemon balm (melissa), both of which are natural antihistamines and useful for treating allergy-related breathing problems. Camomile has a calming, anti-inflammatory effect and is especially useful for over-sensitivity. Lemon balm, too, can calm the antispasmodic "reflex reaction" that happens in allergic conditions.

compresses

A cool compress is best for inflamed conditions. To make one, you need a piece of soft, clean cotton and a small bowl of water. Add 4–6 drops of oil to the water and stir to disperse the oils. Soak the cloth in the water, squeeze it lightly and place over the upper back or chest. Leave it in position for about 30–45 minutes, making sure you stay warm and comfortable.

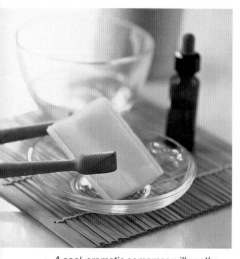

▲ A cool, aromatic compress will soothe inflamed and painful sinuses.

YEAR-ROUND ALLERGIES
Allergic rhinitis is an allergic condition that persists throughout the year with the same sort of symptoms as hay fever – watery eyes, sneezing and a runny nose. It can be caused by a variety of triggers, the most common ones being house dust, pet fur, artificial perfumes and chemicals.

20

steam inhalation

A steam inhalation is one of the most beneficial treatments for clearing the airways of congestion and encouraging better breathing. Adding certain essential oils can make it even more effective.

Eucalyptus has a highly distinctive, camphorous scent that seems to have an almost magical effect on blocked sinuses and "heavy" breathing. Native to Australia, eucalyptus has a powerful antiseptic action, making it a good choice as a preventative measure against winter colds and flu, which can make life especially difficult for asthma sufferers.

Most people either love or loathe the scent of tea tree, which is sharp and slightly pungent. Tea tree is also known for its strong antiseptic properties and is especially valuable for relieving catarrh and sinusitis as well as protecting against colds and flu. Similarly, rosemary has a camphorous, refreshing aroma that is also useful for warding off colds and flu as well as easing the tight, "full-up" feeling across the chest associated with bronchitis and asthma.

steamy aroma

Inhalation is the quickest way for essential oil molecules to be absorbed into the body. To make a steam inhalation, fill a basin with 600ml (1 pt/2½ cups) of boiling water and add 2–3 drops of essential oil. Sit over the bowl making a "tent" with a towel around your head and inhale the vapours. If you experience any discomfort, stop immediately – sometimes, asthmatics cannot tolerate this form of treatment as it can feel claustrophobic and induce feelings of anxiety and panic.

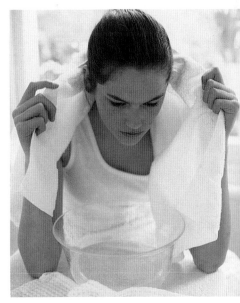

▲ An oil-enriched steam inhalation can help ease congestion.

21 soothing chest rub

A chest rub is an old-fashioned remedy for helping to clear congestion from the lungs. It is easy to make your own aromatic rub, using a base cream and essential oils.

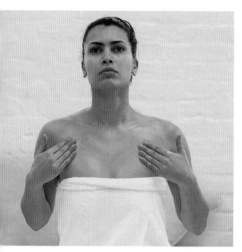

▲ Using a gentle but firm pressure, rub a little aromatic cream into your upper chest. The essential oils, combined with a soothing massage, will have a therapeutic effect.

For thick, chesty coughs and bronchitis, some of the most useful oils are frankincense, myrrh and benzoin. All have a calming, expectorant action on the body.

Frankincense is one of the most useful essential oils for the respiratory system; it slows and deepens the breathing and also has a calming, comforting effect. Both myrrh and benzoin (resinoid) have especially strong expectorant properties. Benzoin has a rich, vanilla-like aroma and is one of the main ingredients in "Friar's Balsam" cough mixture, a traditional syrup for easing chesty coughs. Myrrh also has a balsamic, slightly musty aroma and is especially helpful for clearing excess mucus. It has a slightly sedating effect and is good to use last thing at night.

All these oils are resinous and thus quite "heavy" fragrances, so you may prefer to use one or two of them as a base and combine with light-smelling oils such as lavender, herbaceous scents such as thyme or camphorous aromas such as eucalyptus, all of which have an affinity with the respiratory system.

aromatic cream recipe

To make a chest rub, add 5 drops of essential oil to a 50ml jar of unscented base cream. Blend the oil(s) into the cream using a toothpick or the handle of a teaspoon. Rub the cream well into your chest before going to bed, using a soothing circular stroke. The cream will keep for 2–3 months.

22 lavender sinus massage

Lavender is probably the most versatile essential oil. It has a gentle, balancing action on the body and a refreshing, distinctive scent. Use it to clear blocked and painful sinuses.

Inflammation of the sinus area around the nose and/or eyes causes chronic congestion, catarrh, headaches and breathing difficulties. It is a painful condition that is exacerbated by allergic reactions or colds. Lavender is a natural analgesic (pain-killer) and also has antiseptic and antibiotic properties. Its healing, soothing qualities make it ideal for treating painful sinus problems.

quick-fix self-massage sequence

To make a massage oil mixture, add 4–5 drops lavender essential oil to 30ml (2 tbsp) sweet almond oil, and stir to blend. As you massage your face, take great care to ensure that you keep the oil well away from your eyes.

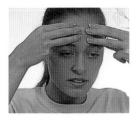

1 Place your hands just above the mid-point between the eyebrows. Make small circles with your fingers, working your way across the forehead. Apply gentle pressure.

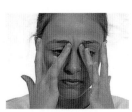

2 Place your middle fingers either side of the nose. Breathe in, and on the out-breath press firmly for a few seconds, then release. Repeat three times.

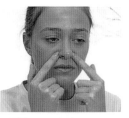

3 With your index fingers on either side of your nose, press gently, holding and releasing. Repeat three times. This is an important pressure point for opening up the sinuses.

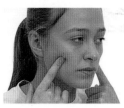

4 Draw your fingers along the cheekbones applying pressure strokes. Then use your thumbs to make small circular movements along this line.

23 healing bath oils

Essential oils in the bath have a two-fold effect: they are absorbed through the skin while their aroma is inhaled, having an immediate effect on the respiratory system.

Sandalwood is widely used in Ayurvedic medicine, the ancient healing system of India, where it has many medicinal uses, especially in the treatment of bacterial infections. In the West, aromatherapists use sandalwood to treat many different conditions, including chronic bronchitis and respiratory disorders that are characterized by a dry, irritating and tickly cough. Some people prefer the scent of sandalwood to the more floral fragrances. Alternatively, marjoram is effective for respiratory conditions. According to Culpeper, the 17th-century English herbalist, it "helpeth all diseases of the chest which hinder the freeness of breathing". It seems particularly effective with asthma, bronchitis and colds, and for relaxing spasmodic, tickly coughs. It can also loosen mucus and, if used at the early onset of a cold, may prevent it turning into a nasty chest infection that is much harder to shift.

essential oil bathing

Both marjoram and sandalwood have a sedative effect, and are thus good choices to use in a bedtime bath. To use essential oils in the bath, run the water first and then add 4–5 drops of oil. Swirl the water to disperse the oils. For maximum benefit, soak in the water for at least ten minutes.

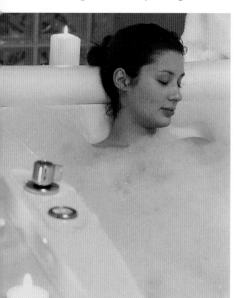

◄ An aromatic sandalwood bath can ease a dry cough and promote a good night's sleep. Breathe deeply as you soak to experience the full healing effect of the essential oil.

24 homeopathy

Based on a "like cures like" principle, homeopathy stimulates the body's naturally well-balanced self-healing mechanism. Homeopathy offers a range of remedies to help breathing disorders.

Conventional science has as yet no plausible explanation for homeopathic medicine. The remedies are prepared from plant, animal and mineral substances that are diluted to such an extent that no molecules of the original substance remain. Practitioners claim, however, that homeopathy is a form of vibrational or energy medicine: that what remains in the remedy is the "energetic blueprint" of the original substance, which works on the body's subtle energy system, rather than directly on the physical body.

A homeopathic remedy is selected by matching it to your particular physical, mental and emotional symptoms. This list will help you match a remedy to your symptoms. Take a 6c potency pill, three times a day, until your symptoms improve.

first-aid for hay fever and rhinitis
ALLIUM CEPA: burning nasal discharge and watery eyes.
ARSENICUM: burning eyes with tears that feel hot; sneezing brings no relief.
EUPHRASIA: profuse runny nose which blocks at night; eyes feel sore.

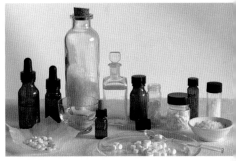

▲ Homeopathic remedies are highly diluted. They are available in pill and tincture form.

first-aid for sinusitis
HEPAR SULPH: painful swelling of the nasal cavities with yellow mucus.
NAT MUR: profuse watery discharge; sneezing, frontal headache.
SILICA: dry blocked nose, severe headache with bouts of sneezing; worse for cold, better for warmth.

first-aid for coughs
BRYONIA: dry, hacking cough, made worse by changes in temperature.
IPECAC: spasmodic cough with rattly mucus on the chest.
PHOSPHORUS: hoarse voice, dry tickly cough and a tight feeling like a band around the chest.

25 reiki healing

Originating in Japan, reiki is a form of spiritual healing that is very gentle and non-invasive. It is particularly useful for breathing problems associated with panic and anxiety.

In Japanese, "rei-ki" can be translated as "universal-life energy". A treatment involves channelling this cosmic energy, or light, to where it is most needed in the body. To give a treatment, visualize a stream of golden light entering the crown of your head, pouring through your body and constantly flowing out through your hands as you work.

treating the upper chest

When we work on the upper chest area we are also connecting with the energies of the heart. A shallow breathing pattern and tension in the upper chest may be associated with emotional hurts and disappointments that have become "locked" in the body. Channelling reiki to this area can help to release these in a way that is comforting and soothing.

Sitting at your partner's head, place your hands in an inverted "V" position at the top of the chest. Holding this position soothes and relaxes tension and is also a tonic for the lungs. It can help clear mucus from the airways and is effective for asthma sufferers and smokers.

easing a cold

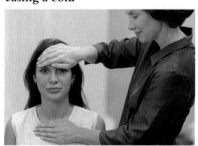

1 To treat a stuffy, blocked-up nose and painful sinuses, place one hand on the upper chest and the other across your partner's forehead.

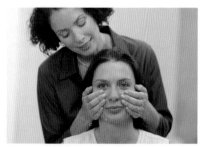

2 Follow this by positioning your hands across your partner's face, with your index and middle fingers touching the cheekbones.

26

colour therapy

Bringing colour energies into the body is another way of rebalancing body and soul. It is particularly useful for breathing problems with a strong emotional component.

Colour is light vibrating at a particular frequency, with colours at the red end of the spectrum having a lower frequency than those at the blue end. Each band of colour has different qualities and associations that can be used for healing. This visualization is a simple but effective way of bringing the healing power of colour into your body – it can also indicate which colour energies you are most in need of absorbing.

BETTER BREATHING WITH COLOUR
red: "emotional" asthma characterized by insecurity and nervousness.
orange: clears mucus; therapeutic for hay fever.
yellow: strengthens resistance to allergic reactions and colds.
green: expansive; relaxes tense chest muscles; useful for asthma and other respiratory problems.
blue and indigo: calms over-excited or agitated states; useful for desensitizing allergic reactions.
violet: speeds up the body's healing processes; balancing.

rainbow breathing

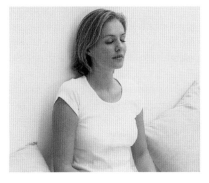

1 Sit with eyes closed in a comfortable position. Relax and allow your breathing to slow and settle.

2 Imagine the air around you is a rich, deep red. As you breathe in, imagine that your whole body fills with red energy. Continue breathing in the red light, then imagine breathing it out through your feet into the earth.

3 Repeat step two, this time imagining the air is a vibrant, warm orange colour. When you have finished with orange, continue with the other colours of the rainbow: yellow, green, blue, indigo and violet.

chakra balancing

Disturbances in breathing are linked to imbalances in the chakra system. Working on the chakras of the upper body can help restore healthy breathing.

The chakras are subtle energy centres that run up the front and back of the body. Each chakra corresponds to different organs of the body and has colour and gemstone associations.

chakras of the upper body
The heart chakra is located at the centre of the chest and is related to the heart, lungs and arms. Its colour correspondence is green and its gemstone is rose quartz. The ears, nose and mouth are under the

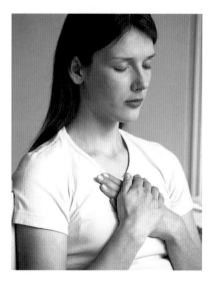

influence of the throat chakra, which also deals with communication and creative self-expression. Its colour is blue and its stone is turquoise. The brow chakra or "third eye" is in the centre of the forehead and relates to the pineal gland, which influences our mood and behaviour. Its colour is indigo and the gemstone is lapis lazuli.

rebalancing the chakras
For asthma and chronic chest complaints, concentrate on the heart chakra. For colds, hay fever and allergic rhinitis, focus on the throat chakra; and for sinus problems, work on the third eye.

Sit in a comfortable position with your eyes closed. Place your hands over the corresponding chakra. Take a deep breath into the area and hold the breath for as long as feels comfortable; then breathe out. If you want to use gemstones and/or colour, either visualize the colour or hold the appropriate stone, or a crystal, over the chakra as you breathe.

◄ Focussing on the heart chakra can have a soothing effect on the respiratory system.

28

flower essences

Some breathing disorders have a strong mental and emotional component. Flower essences are useful for treating negative emotional states and restoring balance.

In many parts of the world, flower essences have been used in healing for thousands of years. In the West, the Bach flower essences were developed by Dr Edward Bach in the 1920s after Bach found that his mood was altered in different ways by certain plants.

the Bach flowers

Bach flower essences can be useful for breathing problems that have a strong emotional component or are made worse by stress, such as asthma or hyperventilation (panic attacks).

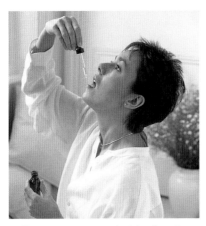

▲ Flower essences may be taken in water or undiluted. Take 2–3 drops.

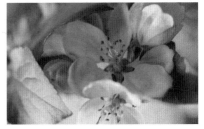

▲ The cleansing action of crab apple can help clear mucus from the airways.

Select a remedy by matching your symptoms to the remedy description.

Bach flower remedy selector

ASPEN: fearful of the dark, of dying, of the future.

CRAB APPLE: cleanser and detoxifier.

IMPATIENS: tense and irritable, often with a headache.

MIMULUS: anxious and fearful for known causes.

WHITE CHESTNUT: a mind that will not switch off.

OLIVE: mentally and physically drained and exhausted.

ROCK ROSE: severe panic; terror, fright, hysteria.

RESCUE REMEDY: multi-purpose first-aid remedy for shock and panic.

29 fortifying garlic

Since ancient times, garlic has been valued as a powerful herbal medicine for strengthening the respiratory system and building immunity. It is an effective preventative measure.

In Traditional Chinese Medicine (TCM), garlic was prescribed to keep coughs and colds at bay, while it was used in ancient Greek and Roman times to treat respiratory infections. In more recent times, Louis Pasteur, the 19th-century French chemist, discovered that garlic had antiseptic properties and it was first used to treat TB in the early 20th century. In fact, before antibiotics were developed, garlic was widely used to treat all kinds of infections.

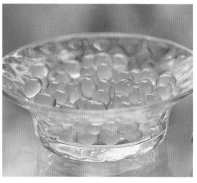

▲ A convenient way of taking garlic is as odourless capsules or pearls. Take 1–3 a day.

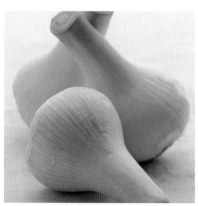

▲ Garlic is a powerful herbal remedy for many kinds of infections, but its ability to help clear mucus makes it especially effective at combatting chest ailments.

Garlic can be strengthening and revitalizing, and because its volatile oil is largely excreted through the lungs, it has a particular affinity with the respiratory system.

Ideally, it is best eaten raw – in ancient Egypt, slaves were fed several cloves of garlic a day to keep them strong and healthy. However, many people dislike garlic's pungent taste and odour, in which case try it lightly stir-fried, making sure it does not go brown as this will give it a bitter taste. Alternatively, garlic capsules are widely available; take 1–3 daily as a preventative measure.

30 protective echinacea

Purple coneflower, or echinacea, is one of the most powerful medicines in the Native American tradition. The plant has many healing properties and a strong affinity with the respiratory system.

Inspired by the plant's spiky central cone, the name echinacea is derived from the Greek *echinos*, meaning hedgehog. Echinacea can help the body fight off infections by boosting the immune system. While Native Americans have used echinacea to treat all kinds of illnesses, including poisonous bites, wounds and fevers, research has shown that it is also helpful for chronic infections, problems related to the upper respiratory tract, and allergies.

As a herbal remedy, echinacea is available in tincture or capsule form in good health stores and pharmacies.

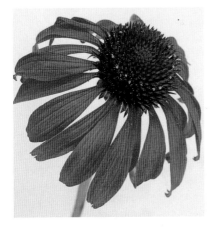

To treat colds and upper respiratory tract infections, take 2.5ml/½ tsp tincture diluted in water, or a 500mg capsule, three times a day. As a preventative measure, to strengthen the immune system, take 2.5ml/½ tsp tincture or a 500mg capsule once a day. Echinacea should not be taken for more than two or three weeks at a time, and should be avoided when pregnant or breastfeeding.

As well as boosting the immune system, echinacea can act as a tonic to balance it. Allergic conditions – such as hay fever, rhinitis and allergic asthma - are triggered when the immune system overreacts to a stimulant, such as pollen, dust or fur, or certain foods and chemicals. Not realizing these substances are harmless, the body mounts a full-scale defence against them, producing symptoms such as wheezing, sneezing, congestion, watery eyes, a runny nose. Echinacea can help to suppress this reaction and stabilize the immune system.

◀ *For colds, flu, bronchitis and other types of infection, echinacea gives the immune system a tremendous boost.*

31 healing herb tinctures

The antiseptic and tonic action of thyme makes it a useful immunity-booster as well as an effective remedy for chest infections, such as pleurisy, bronchitis and whooping cough.

Culpeper, the 17th-century English herbalist, described thyme as a strengthener of the lungs and one of the best remedies for whooping cough. Thyme is a powerful expectorant and useful for treating viral chest infections.

Many herbs contain active ingredients that are not easily extracted by water or are destroyed by heat. A tincture solves these problems as well as preserving the extract. A tincture is an extract of a herb in a mixture of alcohol and water, normally 25 per cent alcohol strength, with the alcohol preserving

the medicine for two years or more. As tinctures are concentrated extracts, they should only be used for short periods of time. Take 5ml/1tsp of tincture three times a day, diluted in water or fresh juice.

preparing a thyme tincture
200g/7oz dried or 300g/11oz
    fresh thyme
750ml/1¼ pints/3 cups water
250ml/8fl oz/1 cup vodka

Chop up the herb and place in a large glass storage jar. Pour on the alcohol and water, seal the jar and leave in a cool place for two weeks. Shake the jar occasionally. Pour the mixture through a piece of muslin (cheesecloth) into a clean jar or bottle, seal well and store in a cool place.

▲ Tinctures are concentrated medicinal extracts and should be used sparingly.

CAT'S THYME
A herb known as cat's thyme or *Marum verum* has been used as a form of snuff. It is said to reduce inflammation of the nasal passages and is a useful remedy for nasal polyps and snoring.

32

nettle and elderflower tisane

A tisane is a good way to use the more delicate parts of plants, especially their leaves and flowers. Try a combination of nettles and elderflower for a range of breathing disorders.

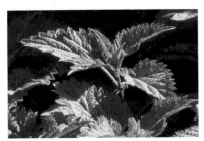

▲ Fresh nettle tops can be cooked and eaten as a vegetable or made into a tisane.

The warming action of nettles makes them useful for colds, while their anti-inflammatory and anti-allergic properties make them especially useful for asthma and hay fever. As well as being made into a drink, nettle leaves can also be lightly cooked and eaten as a vegetable. Eating cooked nettle tops in the springtime is said to be an effective detoxifier, helping to rid the body of excess phlegm accumulated during the winter.

Elderflowers can also be helpful for respiratory problems, including asthma and colds. Elderflower remedies have a relaxing and decongesting effect on the bronchi, thereby reducing muscle spasm and helping to expel excess mucus. They also have a toning effect on the mucous linings of the nose and throat and increase resistance to infection.

tisane recipe

Taken regularly for a few months before the hay fever season, a nettle and elderflower tisane can really help. It can also help to reduce catarrh, so is useful for colds, bronchitis and asthma. To make a tisane, pour a cup of near-boiling water on 5ml/1 tsp each of fresh chopped leaves and blossoms, or 2.5ml/½ tsp each of the dried herbs. Leave for 10–15 minutes. Strain and drink three times a day.

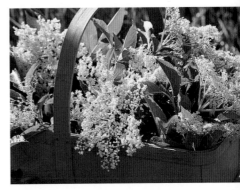

▲ Elderflowers can be used to make a remedy for respiratory problems.

33 easy-breathing tea

Herbal teas are an easy and convenient way of using herbal medicines. Some of the best herbal treatments for chest and sinus problems are yarrow, elderflowers, peppermint and elecampane.

One of nature's best "lung herbs" is elecampane, which is particularly useful for treating chronic bronchitis and bronchial asthma. Elecampane has a powerful anti-inflammatory and soothing action. It also reduces mucus secretions, is a powerful expectorant and stimulates the whole of the immune system.

Another plant known for its anti-inflammatory qualities is yarrow, it also has antiseptic, antispasmodic and anti-allergic properties, which make it useful for treating hay fever. It also acts as a tonic to the nervous system, and can help calm the irritated, anxious states associated with some breathing problems.

Elderflowers can be used to soothe an irritated respiratory system, while peppermint has invigorating antiseptic properties and is useful for clearing blocked sinuses and treating chesty colds. The antispasmodic action of peppermint makes it useful for easing bronchial spasm in asthma and for calming tension and anxiety; it is also a good warming herb for relieving winter colds and chills.

easy-breathing recipe

This recipe uses a combination of yarrow, peppermint, elecampane and elderflower in a tea that encourages the airways to open while protecting and invigorating the immune system. To make the tea you will need 2.5ml/½ tsp of each herb per 250ml/8fl oz/1 cup of near-boiling water. For fresh flowers and leaves, double the quantity of each herb. Add the herbs to the hot water and leave to steep for 5–10 minutes. Strain off the liquid and drink two or three times a day. Sweeten with honey to taste.

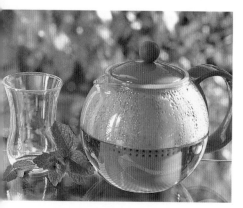

▲ It is easy to make your own herbal teas.
Simply add the herb to hot water and infuse.

34

camomile and eyebright infusion

In cases of hay fever and allergic rhinitis, camomile and eyebright will treat physical and mental symptoms. The plants may be used separately or together in an infusion.

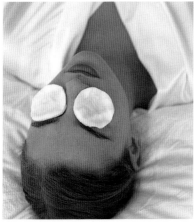

◀ To relieve the itchy, sore red eyes associated with hay fever, soak cotton pads in a camomile and eyebright infusion.

There are two main varieties of camomile, Roman and German, with similar properties, but it is German camomile (Matricaria recutica) that is especially useful for hay fever and allergic asthma. This is due to some of its key constituents, which have a strong antispasmodic action, relieving irritability and promoting calm. Research has shown that camomile is also a natural antihistamine, giving it an anti-allergic effect.

As its name suggests, eyebright (or euphrasia as it is sometimes known) can be helpful for treating allergic conditions such as hay fever and rhinitis that involve itchy, red and watery eyes. Eyebright has a tightening effect on the mucous membranes of the eyes and reduces inflammation. It also counters catarrh, making it useful for clearing the sinuses and the nasal passages. However, it is not recommended for a stuffy, blocked-up nose, but only for conditions where mucus is watery, profuse and free-flowing.

making an infusion

To make an infusion, pour a cup of near-boiling water on the herbs – using 5ml/1 tsp of each fresh chopped herb, or 2.5ml/½ tsp of dried herb. Leave to stand for 10–15 minutes, strain and use as required.

A camomile and eyebright infusion can be used in two ways: first, as a tea to be taken two or three times a day; and secondly, by soaking pads of cotton wool in a cooled infusion and placing them on the eyelids to soothe sore, irritated eyes.

35 vitamin A

One of the most important vitamins for helping to maintain a healthy respiratory system is vitamin A. It guards against infection and helps protect the lungs against pollution.

Vitamin A can be stored by the body and need not be replenished every day. It occurs in two forms: first as preformed vitamin A, or retinol, and second as provitamin A, or carotene. The former is found only in foods of animal origin, while the second is provided by both plant and animal-derived foods.

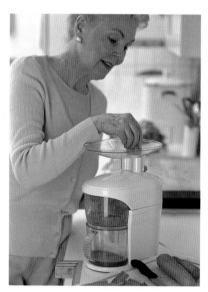

▲ Carrots provide a versatile source of vitamin A. For maximum benefit, enjoy them raw, in salads or as a fresh juice.

Some of the best natural sources of vitamin A are carrots, fish liver oil, liver, green and yellow vegetables, eggs, milk and dairy products. If you eat plenty of these foods you will provide your body with adequate vitamin A. However, some breathing problems are exacerbated by eating too many dairy products and eggs. It is also worth bearing in mind that foods lose their vitamins once they have been picked and stored, and that non-organic varieties may also contain traces of pesticides or antibiotics.

If you suffer from a serious respiratory condition, such as asthma, bronchitis, pleurisy or emphysema, you would probably do well to take a vitamin A supplement, at least until the symptoms improve. Supplements are usually available in two forms, one that is derived from fish oils – such as cod-liver oil – and another that is water-dispersible and recommended for anyone who has trouble tolerating oil, such as those suffering from oily skin, for example. A typical daily dose is 10,000 IU, but always check the label on the container to find out how many capsules to take.

36 B vitamins

The B vitamins play an essential role in more than 60 metabolic reactions. B vitamins are particularly helpful for breathing problems that are stress-related, such as asthma and hyperventilation.

There are more than ten members of B vitamin complex, and collectively, B vitamins are particularly involved in energy production and are probably best known for their effect on the nervous system.

Also known as the anti-stress vitamin, B5 (or pantothenic acid) has been found to be particularly useful for treating stress, but of all the B vitamins, B6 (or pyridoxine) is probably the most important one. It is involved in more bodily functions than almost any other nutrient and affects both physical and mental health. B6 is an immunity booster and has an affinity with the nervous system, making it helpful for treating allergies and asthma. However, the B vitamins generally work best when taken as a complex, as their effect is synergistic: in other words, the action of one enhances that of another.

Foods that are good natural sources of B vitamins include wheat germ, brewer's yeast, brown rice, fish, liver, eggs, milk and cheese as well as cabbage and avocados.

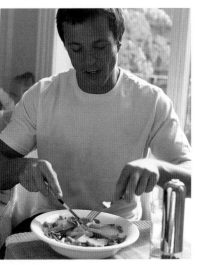

▲ Avocados provide plenty of B vitamins – add them to salads and sandwiches.

If your breathing problems are stress-related, it may help to take a B vitamin complex supplement, as B vitamins are used up more quickly when you are stressed. Look for a "time release" supplement, which means that the vitamins are contained in a special formula that will slowly release the nutrients over a seven- to eight-hour time period. A high-potency dose would be around 350mg a day.

Increase your intake of vitamin C and eat plenty of fresh fruit.

Vitamin C is a natural antihistamine and will help to keep hay fever and allergies under control.

38 quercetin

A compound that is found in apples, tea, onions and red wine, quercetin is said to be helpful for allergy-related problems such as allergic rhinitis, asthma and hay fever.

Quercetin is a member of a large group of water-soluble plant compounds called flavonoids. It acts as an antihistamine, so it is helpful for calming allergic reactions, and it also has useful anti-inflammatory and antioxidant properties.

Quercetin may help to alleviate the symptoms of asthma, allergies and hay fever in some sufferers. Good natural sources include apples, raspberries, red grapes, citrus fruits, onions and leafy green vegetables. Alternatively, red wine and black and green tea also contain this flavonoid. Quercetin is also available as a supplement, available in good health stores and pharmacies: the recommended dose is 400mg two or three times a day.

WHAT ARE ALLERGIES?
An allergic reaction is a response mounted by the immune system to a certain food, inhalant (airborne substance), or chemical. Special immune cells called "mast cells" release histamine and other chemicals in order to destroy what the body perceives as a harmful substance. These chemicals cause inflammation and an increase in lymph fluid, and act as a signal for more mast cells to join in.

A typical allergic attack starts with itching in the nose and eyes, followed by watering of the eyes and nose as the body tries to flush out its invaders. Sneezing often comes next – an attempt to remove them more forcibly.

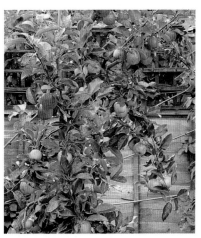

▲ Studies have linked eating five or more apples (rich in quercetin) a week with improved lung function and a lower risk of respiratory diseases such as asthma, bronchitis and emphysema.

39 zinc

A powerful immunity-booster, zinc is an essential mineral that is required for more than 200 enzyme activities within the body. It can help protect against colds and allergies.

Zinc protects the immune system, and is vital for normal cell division and function, yet many of us are zinc-deficient. Frequent colds, a poor sense of taste or smell and feeling run-down are signs of a deficiency. Stress, sweating – through vigorous exercise for instance – smoking and high tea, coffee, alcohol and refined food consumption all deplete zinc reserves.

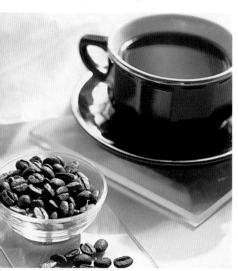

▲ Coffee may have a tempting aroma, but it is worth remembering that it depletes your body's zinc reserves.

The best natural sources include red meat and shellfish, particularly mussels, oysters and crabmeat. Liver and dried brewer's yeast are also high in zinc and other sources include pumpkin seeds, eggs and wholegrain products. Choose organic foods where possible, because modern farming methods mean that many foods are grown in soils that are low in vital minerals, and trace elements such as zinc are lost through processing methods.

Asthmatics and those suffering from chronic chest problems are particularly vulnerable to colds and flu. To protect yourself and strengthen immunity, it is worth considering taking a zinc supplement of between 15 and 20mg a day with a glass of orange juice (vitamin C aids zinc absorption). Zinc supplements should not be taken on an empty stomach because they may make you feel sick. Zinc lozenges are also available for colds and sore throats: it seems that zinc may have a direct effect on the cold viruses in the mouth, nose and throat and stop them from multiplying.

40

say "no" to...

What we eat has a direct bearing on our health and fitness. Certain foods are known to aggravate breathing problems so it may help to avoid them and look for healthier options.

The number of people suffering from asthma and allergies has risen dramatically in the last 50 years. During this time our diet has changed quite radically, and our consumption of refined and highly processed foods, that are far from their natural state, has increased dramatically.

what to avoid

Research has shown that refined carbohydrates depress the immune system within one hour of being consumed. These include all products containing white flour or sugar – bread, biscuits, cake and pasta, as well as sweets and chocolate. For a tasty snack, eat fresh fruit, nuts or cereal bars instead. It may also be that a diet high in animal fats reduces the immune system's efficiency, while sugar and wheat are another two foodstuffs that weaken immunity, and also contribute to the formation of mucus. Honey is a natural alternative to sugar, and if you want to avoid wheat, you can try eating more of other grains such as millet, rye, or rice. Rice cakes make a low-calorie, healthy alternative to bread.

Milk, eggs and cheese are a good source of calcium but may encourage mucus production. Try substituting calcium-enriched soya milk instead of cow's milk, or you may find your body tolerates goat's or sheep's milk better.

Finally, foods that contain artificial colourings, flavourings, preservatives can aggravate asthma and allergies and are best avoided.

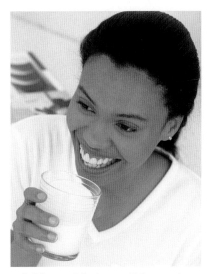

▲ Calcium-enriched soya milk is a good substitute for cow's milk as it helps to ensure you are getting the calcium you need.

41

say "yes" to...

The healing power of food was recognized by Hippocrates, the "father of medicine", more than 2000 years ago. And there are certain foods that can help to support better breathing.

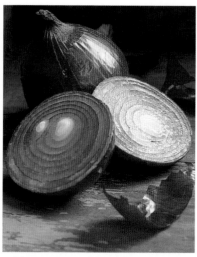

▲ *Onions have a long tradition as a healing food for asthma and respiratory problems.*

To keep your body healthy it is important to eat a varied and balanced diet, including as much fresh, organic produce as possible. Dark green vegetables such as broccoli, cabbage and spinach, as well as root vegetables such as carrots, turnips and onions, are all good for respiratory problems. Oily fish, such as salmon, mackerel and herring, help the immune system, while millet is a particularly low-allergenic food, and brown rice is known for its calming effect on the nervous system.

healing onions

As well as having cleansing and detoxifying properties, onions are a natural antibiotic and antiseptic and have an antispasmodic effect. It is for these reasons that onions are a traditional treatment for asthma, as they are believed to reduce bronchial spasm.

quick-fix onion soup

2 large onions
15ml/1 tbsp sunflower oil
1 litre/1¾ pints/4 cups stock
   (chicken or vegetable)
fresh thyme
½ tsp yeast extract
black pepper

Peel and chop the onions. Heat the oil in a heavy pan and soften the onions, taking care not to brown them. Add the stock, thyme, yeast extract and pepper. Bring to the boil and simmer gently for 15–20 minutes. Pour the soup into bowls and serve.

42

check it out...

Smoking aside, allergies and intolerances are probably the most common single cause of respiratory problems. Adverse food reactions are linked to many of these problems.

True food allergies are potentially life-threatening, but are relatively rare. Food intolerances, however, are more common, but they are often difficult to detect. Many people believe they are linked to allergies.

COMMON FOOD INTOLERANCES
cereals: wheat is the main problem, although rye is another culprit.
cow's milk: dairy products such as cheese and butter made from cow's milk.
shellfish: mussels, prawns, crab, lobster, scallops.
eggs: an egg allergy is often found in asthmatics.
yeast: found in bread, fermented products such as wine and beer, and yeast extract spreads.
nuts: especially walnuts and hazelnuts.
food additives: these include sulphites (preservatives found in many foods and difficult to isolate); tartrazine (a yellow colouring); MSG (monosodium glutamate; a flavour-enhancer that is widely used in Chinese cooking).

the elimination diet

The best way to check for a food intolerance is by eliminating suspect foods from your diet to see if your symptoms improve. This can be tricky as many common triggers are found in a huge variety of everyday foods, so you will need to check the labels of everything you buy. Cut out all the common triggers for a couple of weeks and keep to a fairly plain diet until your symptoms improve. You may then reintroduce the food groups, one by one; if your symptoms don't return after two or three days, that food or food group is probably safe for you.

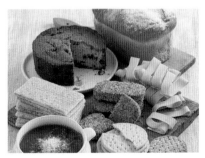

▲ *A wheat intolerance is quite common. Wheat-containing foods include bread, cake, pasta, wheat, cereals, biscuits and processed soups.*

43

body cleanse

When breathing problems are associated with thick catarrh that just won't seem to shift, then a detox or body cleanse may be what is required. A fresh juice fast is a good way to start.

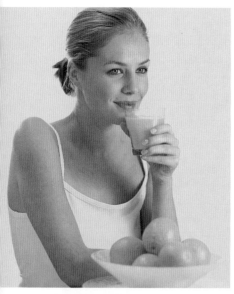

▲ *Detoxing with fresh juices gives your digestive system a rest and can help clear mucus from the body.*

The bacteria that populate the colon and the small intestine have an important part to play in health, including the health of the respiratory system. In fact, it is estimated that 70 per cent of our lymphatic defence system, essential for fighting infection, lies in the bowel wall.

The delicate balance of our intestinal environment can be upset by many things, including stress, eating the wrong foods and taking synthetic drugs. Allergies and the over-production of mucus are signs that the body's internal balance is out of kilter. A body cleanse or detox can give your body a chance to rest and repair itself.

one-day detox

Try a one-day fresh fruit or vegetable juice detox. Juices boost the immune system, help restore the body's delicate pH balance, are easy to digest, and are packed with energy – they also taste great. When juice-fasting, choose a time when you are able to relax and take care of yourself. Expect to feel worse to begin with – it's a sign that your body is throwing out toxins.

carrot and apple cleanse

To make enough for one serving, take three carrots, scrubbed and trimmed, and a couple of apples, washed and cut into quarters. Using a juice extractor, juice the carrots and apples and pour into a glass. Drink by sipping slowly.

Add a piece of cinnamon and a couple of cloves to a hot ginger and lemon tea – this spicy drink will unclog your airways and leave you room to breathe.

45 in the workplace

At work we are subjected to a range of potential "allergens" that can be problematic for asthma and allergies. These include chemicals, dust and electromagnetic pollution.

A typical office contains a vast array of electronic equipment, including computers, laser printers, scanners and photocopiers, as well as telephones – both land lines and mobiles. Research shows that the electromagnetic radiation emitted by such equipment interferes with the body's electromagnetic field and may be linked to health problems and a general weakening of our immunity.

If you suffer breathing problems it is particularly important to protect yourself against these potentially harmful influences, as a weakened immune system increases the likelihood of your condition getting worse. Make sure you take regular breaks away from your computer and keep potted plants and quartz crystals near electronic equipment to help absorb the energy waves. Lack of natural light can also be a problem so make sure your work area uses bulbs that simulate natural daylight rather than fluorescent tube lighting.

toxic substances

There are also many environmental toxins. In an office, the laser carbon in photocopiers and printers can trigger an allergic reaction – sneezing, shortness of breath and watery eyes. Make sure you sit as far away from this equipment as possible, and if possible avoid changing the toner cartridge. Chemicals in paint, glue, cleaning products and even felt-tipped pens can also provoke a reaction, while various dusts (from wood or cotton for instance), fumes, gases and aerosol mists or sprays can be extremely damaging.

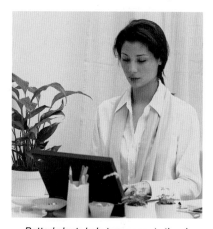

▲ *Potted plants help to oxygenate the air and can absorb some of the negative effects of electromagnetic radiation.*